Exercises for the Neck and Lower Back

A Practical Guide to Strengthening and Stretching

Dr. Sindhu George, DPT

Doctor of Physical Therapy

DISCLAIMER

ISBN 979-8-9873594-0-2 (Paperback)

ISBN 979-8-9873594-1-9 (E-book)

Library of Congress Control Number: 2022921775

For business inquiries ONLY: drgeorge@ptspine.com

TABLE OF CONTENTS

ABOUT THIS BOOK

Dr. George is a licensed physical therapist who has suffered from chronic neck and lower back pain. She developed a system of exercises and stretches that can help in alleviating pain and preventing re-injury. The exercises for the neck and lower back are divided into 3 phases of injury. The exercises are appropriate for each phase based on the pain, strength, and level of function.

The purpose of the exercise and stretching regimen is to stretch and strengthen the muscles around the neck and lower back. The regimen is intended to provide overall strength, stability, and flexibility to prevent re-injury.

In addition, the book also has a chapter on activity modification. These include how to lift objects properly without re-injuring the lower back, sleeping positions to alleviate low back pain, and tips to prevent neck and back pain with everyday activities.

<u>Prior to starting any exercises or stretches in this book, you must be evaluated by a physician to make sure these exercises and stretches are appropriate for you.</u> This book does not replace seeing a physical therapist for physical therapy. This book is meant to be a guide for exercises and stretches.

INTRODUCTION

Neck and back pain are common problems that most people have experienced throughout the course of their lives. The purpose of this book is to educate the average person on how to use exercises to regain strength, flexibility and to prevent re-injury. <u>Prior to starting any exercises in this book, you must be evaluated by a physician to make sure these exercises are appropriate for you.</u> This book does not replace seeing a physical therapist for physical therapy. This book is a practical guide for exercises and stretches.

HOW TO USE THIS BOOK

This book focuses on neck and lower back exercises. Each section of this book is divided into three phases. Prior to each phase of exercise, there is an explanation of the phase, and which muscles are being stretched and strengthened.

When progressing to the next phase of exercise, the explanation of the phase will indicate which exercises are a progressive exercise of the previous phase. If exercises can be performed with no discomfort, previous phase exercise can be discontinued. The purpose of the exercise regimen is to stretch and strengthen all the muscles in the neck and lower back, increase stability and prevent re-injury. Exercising 2-3 times a week with a rest day in between exercise days is recommended.

The first phase is when you are feeling the most pain. During this phase, you must be evaluated and treated by a physician for pain and evaluated to see if this exercise book is appropriate for you. Once you are no longer in pain, you can begin the exercises in the first phase. These exercises are designed to strengthen the muscles in a lying down position to reduce any discomfort. During this phase, please refer to chapters 9 and 10 for tips on how to reduce pain and how to modify activities of daily living.

The second phase has more advanced exercises that are in a seated position. The progression of exercises is intended to increase strength and flexibility. The third and final phase of exercises are in the standing position. The third phase is intended to stretch and strengthen all areas surrounding the neck and lower back. Each phase indicates which muscles are being strengthened. You can adjust exercises within the phases based on your strength and tolerance. Some exercises may be easy, and others can be difficult. This will be dependent on your level of pain and function. The most important thing is to stretch and strengthen the muscles surrounding the neck and lower back to provide stability and prevent re-injury. Creating a checklist to keep track may be helpful.

All exercises and stretches should be performed without pain and discomfort in movement. Discontinue any exercises that cause pain and discomfort. <u>Please seek evaluation with your physician should you experience any pain or not have improvement with use of this book. Neck and lower back pain can also be caused by other serious health conditions that require medical attention and not an exercise regimen.</u>

CHAPTER 1:

INTRODUCTION TO NECK EXERCISES

Introduction to Neck (Cervical Spine) Exercises

The cervical spine (neck) consists of 7 vertebrae. Vertebrae are the bones that hold the weight of the neck. In between the vertebrae are the intervertebral discs. They function as shock absorbers for the cervical spine.

The spinal cord is located inside the vertebrae. The spinal cord in the neck contains nerves that go to the arms. The nerves that go to the arms can get injured in the neck or along the path as they travel into the arms. The spinal cord and nerves can also be pinched by the intervertebral disc being pushed out of position (also known as a disc herniation).

Muscle spasms (knots in the muscle) or tightness can occur in the muscles around the neck and arms. Muscle spasms or tightness in the neck and arms can also increase pain and limit motion. Muscle spasms can decrease flexibility and cause poor posture. Stretching is helpful to increase flexibility and improve posture.

Poor posture (such as hunchback posture) can cause the vertebrae to be in poor alignment. This poor alignment can cause muscle weakness or tightness. When the muscles are weak or tight, there is an increased risk of neck pain or injury. Exercises and stretches are helpful to strengthen weak muscles, stretch tight muscles, improve posture and prevent re-injury.

CHAPTER 2:

NECK FIRST PHASE

Neck First Phase

The First Phase of injury describes the initial injury or pain caused by events such as a fall or car accident. The First Phase of an injury can typically last 1-2 weeks depending on the severity of the injury. The areas that are injured are very sensitive to touch. In addition, swelling and redness may also be seen. During this phase, treatment such as medications, rest and ice may be helpful to decrease pain and prevent further injury. <u>Treatment during initial injury should be underneath a physician's supervision.</u>

The pain associated with the initial injury can be decreased with the above treatment. Gentle massage therapy can be used to decrease muscle tightness. <u>Massage therapy should be initiated after consultation with a physician.</u> Once a person is no longer in pain, then gentle therapeutic exercises can be implemented. Exercises in this phase are performed lying down. Exercises should be performed on a bed and **not** on the floor. When performing exercises be sure to breathe normally. Do not hold your breath.

<u>Before beginning any exercise regimen in this book, it is important to consult your physician and make sure these exercises are appropriate for you.</u> Exercises should not be performed if there is any pain. If there is any pain when exercising, discontinue exercise and see a physician.

Neck First Phase Exercises

Chin Tucks – the purpose of this exercise is to correct poor neck posture and strengthen muscles behind the neck.

Lying Down Bicep Curls – the purpose of this exercise is to strengthen muscles in the arms that are affected by neck injury. It is performed in a lying down position during this phase to decrease strain on the neck.

Lying Down Shoulder Pinches – the purpose of this exercise is to strengthen muscles in between the shoulder blades. This helps improve poor posture and improves alignment of vertebrae. It is performed in a lying down position during this phase to decrease strain on the neck.

Chin Tucks

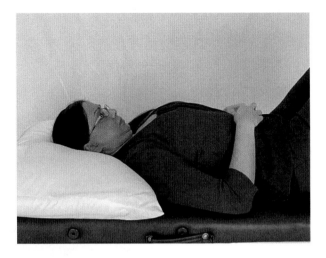

Position 1

Lay down on your back with a pillow under your head. Bend both of your knees.

Tuck your chin into your chest. This will be Position 1. Push your head back into the pillow. This will be

Position 2. Return to Position 1.

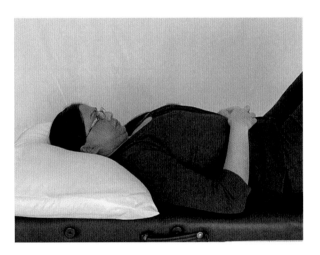

Position 2

When you return to Position 1, this completes one repetition of this exercise. This exercise is used to

strengthen the muscles in the back of your neck. You should feel this exercise in the muscles on the back of

your neck. Repeat exercise 10 times for 1 set. Take a break between sets. Aim to perform 3 sets. Discontinue

if you experience pain.

Lying Down Bicep Curls

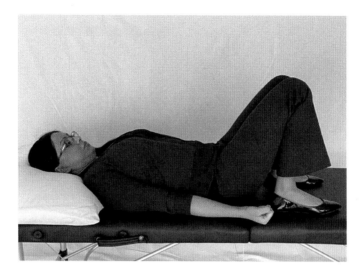

Position 1

Lay down on your back with knees bent. Keep both hands at your sides.

This is Position 1. Bend your elbow by bringing your hands towards your shoulders.

This is Position 2. Return to Position 1.

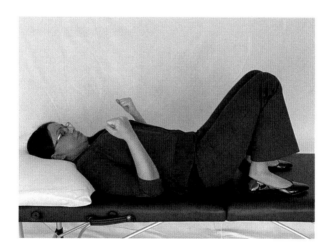

Position 2

When you return to Position 1, this completes one repetition of this exercise. This exercise is used to strengthen the biceps muscles in your arms. You should feel this exercise in the muscles on the front of the upper arms. Repeat exercise 10 times for 1 set. Take a break between sets.

Aim to perform 3 sets. Discontinue if you experience pain.

Lying Down Shoulder Pinches

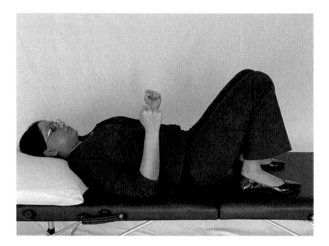

Position 1

Lay down on your back with knees bent. Keep arms at a 90-degree angle to bed.

This is Position 1. With arms at 90-degree angle, push back into bed with elbows. Hold for 3 seconds. This is

Position 2. You should feel this exercise in your upper back between the shoulder blades. Your chest should

rise with this exercise. Return to Position 1.

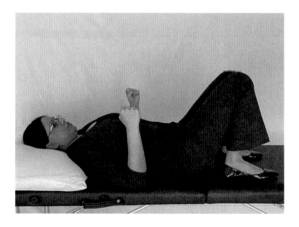

Position 2

When you return to Position 1, this completes one repetition of this exercise. This exercise is to strengthen

the muscles in between the shoulder blades. This will help improve your posture.

Repeat exercise 10 times for 1 set. Take a break between sets. Aim to perform 3 sets.

Discontinue if you experience pain.

CHAPTER 3:

NECK SECOND PHASE

Neck Second Phase

The Second Phase of injury is when the person is not experiencing much pain. However, the person is weak and is at risk for re-injury. The exercises or stretches in this phase should not be performed if there is any pain or discomfort. Continue exercises and stretches from First Phase unless specified below.

Chin tucks – the purpose of this exercise is to correct neck alignment and strengthen the muscles behind the neck. This exercise from Neck First Phase should be continued in Neck Second Phase.

Standing Shoulder Pinches – the purpose of this exercise is to strengthen muscles in between the shoulder blades. This corrects poor posture and improves alignment of the vertebrae. This is a progression of the lying down shoulder pinches in Neck First Phase. This exercise was previously performed lying down. It is now performed standing up. If this exercise can be performed without pain or discomfort, the lying down shoulder pinches can be discontinued.

Shoulder Shrugs – the purpose of this exercise is to strengthen the muscle behind the head and into the top of the shoulder called the upper trapezius. It is important to strengthen this muscle to provide stability for the neck.

Lying Down Bicep Curls – the purpose of this exercise is to strengthen the muscles in the arms that are affected by neck injury. This exercise from Neck First Phase should be continued in the Neck Second Phase.

Standing Shoulder Pinches

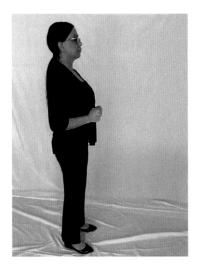

Position 1

Stand tall with arms close to your side. Bend your elbows to 90 degrees. This is Position 1.

Squeeze your shoulder blades together. This is Position 2. Hold for 2-3 seconds. Return to Position 1.

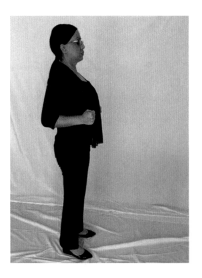

Position 2

When you return to Position 1, this completes one repetition of this exercise.

This exercise is to strengthen the muscles in between the shoulder blades. You should feel the muscles in between your shoulder blades working. This will help improve your posture. Repeat exercise 10 times for 1 set. Take a break between sets. Aim to perform 3 sets. Discontinue if you experience pain.

Shoulder Shrugs

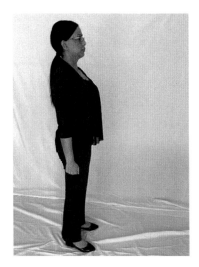

Position 1

Stand up tall and face a mirror. This is Position 1. Shrug your shoulders up and hold for 2-3 seconds. This is Position 2. Return to Position 1.

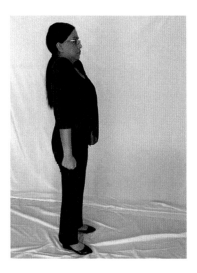

Position 2

When you return to Position 1, this completes one repetition of this exercise.

This exercise strengthens the muscles of the upper shoulder. You should feel this exercise in the muscles in the upper shoulder. Repeat exercise 10 times for 1 set. Take a break between sets. Aim to perform 3 sets. Discontinue if you experience pain.

CHAPTER 4:

NECK THIRD PHASE

Neck Third Phase

The third phase of injury is when the person is not experiencing any pain. The exercises and stretches performed in this phase of injury are designed to improve strength and stability of the surrounding joints. Strengthening the muscles of the shoulders, elbows and wrists will increase neck stability. When first performing exercises for the shoulder, elbow and wrist, do not use weights. As you get stronger, you can start with light weights as tolerated. Increasing neck stability will decrease risk of re-injury. Continue exercises and stretches from First and Second Phases unless specified below.

Shoulder

Active Shoulder Flexion – the purpose of this exercise is to strengthen the muscle in front of the shoulder called the anterior deltoid muscle. Strengthening this muscle can improve shoulder stability.

Shoulder Scaption – the purpose of this exercise is to strengthen the muscle on top of the shoulder called the supraspinatus muscle. Strengthening this muscle can improve shoulder stability.

Shoulder Abduction – the purpose of this exercise is to strengthen the muscle on the side of the shoulder called the middle deltoid muscle. Strengthening this muscle can improve shoulder stability.

Shoulder Extension – the purpose of this exercise is to strengthen the muscle behind the shoulder called the posterior deltoid muscle. Strengthening this muscle can improve shoulder stability.

Elbow

Bicep Curls – discontinue lying down variation of this exercise in Neck First and Second Phases. The purpose of this exercise is to strengthen muscles in front of the upper arm called the biceps muscle. This exercise increases stability for the elbow and shoulder joint.

Triceps Curl Backs - the purpose of this exercise is to strengthen the muscles in the back of the upper arm called the triceps muscle. This exercise increases stability for the elbow and shoulder joint.

Wrist

Wrist Extension - the purpose of this exercise is to strengthen muscles on the top of the forearm (these are collectively called the wrist extensor muscles). This exercise increases stability for the wrist and hand.

Wrist Flexion - the purpose of this exercise is to strengthen muscles on the bottom of the forearm (these are collectively called the wrist flexor muscles). This exercise increases stability for the wrist and hand.

Wrist Radial Deviation - the purpose of this exercise is to strengthen muscles on the thumb side of the forearm. This exercise increases stability for the wrist and hand.

Wrist Ulna Deviation - the purpose of this exercise is to strengthen muscles on the pinky (5th digit) side of the forearm. This exercise increases stability for the wrist and hand.

Wrist Supination - the purpose of this exercise is to strengthen muscles in the forearm that turn the palms up. This exercise increases stability for the wrist and hand.

Wrist Pronation - the purpose of this exercise is to strengthen muscles in the forearm that turn the palms down. This exercise increases stability for the wrist and hand.

Grip Strengthening - the purpose of this exercise is to strengthen muscles in the forearm that help with holding on to objects. This exercise increases stability for the wrist and hand.

Stretches

Wrist Extensor Stretch – the purpose of this stretch is to improve flexibility of the muscles on the top of the forearm. This stretch increases flexibility for the wrist and hand.

Wrist Flexor Stretch – the purpose of this stretch is to improve flexibility of the muscles on the bottom of the forearm. This stretch increases flexibility for the wrist and hand.

Shoulder Stretch #1 and #2 – the purpose of this stretch is to improve flexibility of the muscles of the shoulder. This stretch increases flexibility of the shoulder. **These stretches should not be performed if there is any history of shoulder dislocation or shoulder surgery.**

Corner Pectoralis Stretch – the purpose of this stretch is to improve flexibility of the muscles on the front of the shoulder/chest. This stretch helps improve posture.

Door Post Stretch – this is a progression of the Corner Pectoralis Stretch. If this stretch can be performed without pain, the Corner Pectoralis Stretch can be discontinued. The purpose of this stretch is to improve flexibility of the muscles on the front of the chest/shoulder. This stretch helps improve posture.

Upper Trapezius Stretch - the purpose of this stretch is to improve flexibility of the muscles on the side of neck. This stretch helps improve posture.

Active Shoulder Flexion

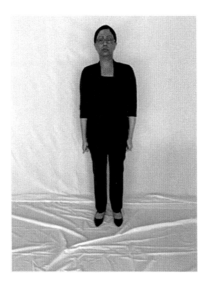

Position 1

Stand up straight and face a mirror. Your arms should be at your side. This is Position 1.

Lift both your arms up in front of you to shoulder level. This is Position 2. Lower your arms to Position 1.

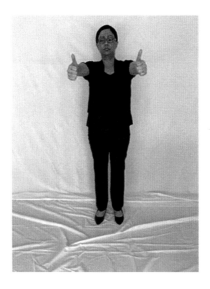

Position 2

When you return to Position 1, this completes one repetition of this exercise. This exercise is used to strengthen the muscles in front of your shoulder. Repeat exercise 10 times for 1 set.

Take a break between sets. Aim to perform 3 sets. Discontinue if you experience pain.

Shoulder Scaption

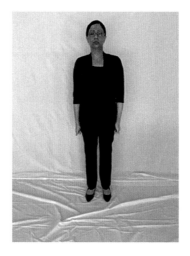

Position 1

Stand up straight and face a mirror. Your arms should be at your side. This is Position 1.

Lift both your arms up in front of you to shoulder level. In this exercise, the arms should be at an angle (like the letter Y). This is Position 2. Lower your arms to Position 1.

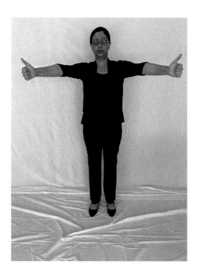

Position 2

When you return to Position 1, this completes one repetition of this exercise. This exercise is used to strengthen the muscles on the top of your shoulder. Repeat exercise 10 times for 1 set.

Take a break between sets. Aim to perform 3 sets. Discontinue if you experience pain

Shoulder Abduction

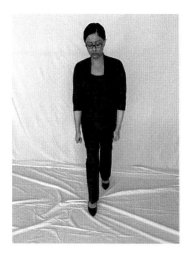

Position 1

Stand up straight and face a mirror. Your arms should be at your side. Place your right foot in front of you.

This is Position 1. Lift both your arms out to the side with thumbs facing up.

Lift your arms just below shoulder level. Do not lift arms over the level of the shoulder. This is Position 2.

Lower your arms to Position 1.

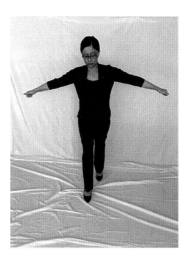

Position 2

When you return to Position 1, this completes one repetition of this exercise. This exercise is to strengthen the muscles on the side of your shoulder. Repeat exercise 10 times for 1 set.

Take a break between sets. Aim to perform 3 sets. Discontinue if you experience pain.

Shoulder Extension

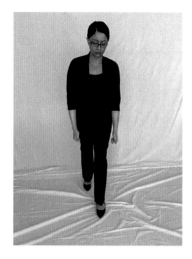

Position 1

Stand up straight and face a mirror. Your arms should be at your side. Place one foot in front of you. This is Position 1. With your arms fully extended at the elbow, bring both of your arms straight back. This is Position 2. Return to Position 1.

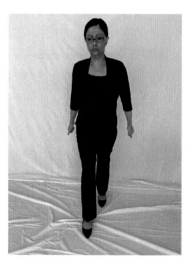

Position 2

When you return to Position 1, this completes one repetition of this exercise. This exercise is to strengthen the muscles on the back of your shoulder. Repeat exercise 10 times for 1 set. Take a break between sets. Aim to perform 3 sets. Discontinue if you experience pain.

Biceps Curls

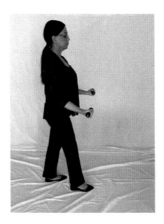

Position 1

Stand up straight and face a mirror. Your arms should be at your side. Place one foot in front of you. Keep your elbows close to your side. Raise your elbows to 90 degrees. This is Position 1. Bend your elbows and bring your hands to your shoulders. This is Position 2.

Return to Position 1.

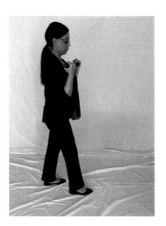

Position 2

When you return to Position 1, this completes one repetition of this exercise.

This exercise is to strengthen the muscles on the front of your arms between the elbow and shoulder.

Repeat exercise 10 times for 1 set. Take a break between sets. Aim to perform 3 sets.

Discontinue if you experience pain.

Triceps Curl Backs

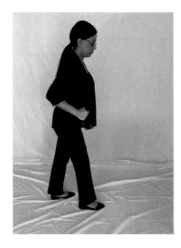

Position 1

Stand up straight and face a mirror. Place one foot in front of you and lean slightly forward.

Keep your elbows close to your side and bend your elbows at a 90-degree angle.

This is Position 1. Extend your arms fully backwards. This is Position 2. Return to Position 1.

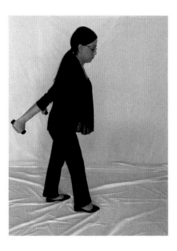

Position 2

When you return to Position 1, this completes one repetition of this exercise. This exercise is to strengthen the muscles on the back of your arms between the elbow and shoulder.

Repeat exercise 10 times for 1 set. Take a break between sets.

Aim to perform 3 sets. Discontinue if you experience pain.

Wrist extension

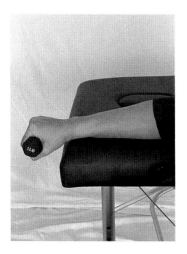

Position 1

Sit down on a chair. Place your forearm on a table or bed, with the wrist hanging off the edge. The wrist should be parallel with the table. This is Position 1. Extend your wrist fully backwards. This is Position 2. Return to Position 1.

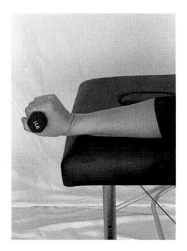

Position 2

When you return to Position 1, this completes one repetition of this exercise. This exercise is to strengthen the muscles on the top of the forearm between the wrist and elbow.

Repeat exercise 10 times for 1 set. Take a break between sets. Aim to perform 3 sets.

Repeat exercise with other hand. Discontinue if you experience pain.

Wrist flexion

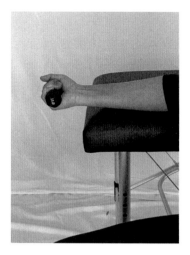

Position 1

Sit down on a chair. Place your forearm on a table or bed, with the wrist hanging off the edge. The palm should be facing upwards. The wrist should be parallel with the table. This is Position 1. Flex your wrist fully towards you. This is Position 2. Return to Position 1.

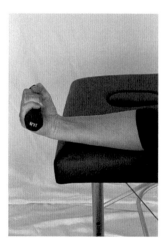

Position 2

When you return to Position 1, this completes one repetition of this exercise.

This exercise is to strengthen the muscles on the bottom side of the forearm between the wrist and elbow. Repeat exercise 10 times for 1 set. Take a break between sets. Aim to perform 3 sets. Repeat exercise with other hand. Discontinue if you experience pain.

Wrist Radial Deviation

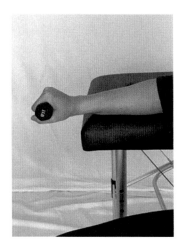

Position 1

Sit down on a chair. Place your forearm on a table or bed, with the wrist hanging off the edge.

The wrist should be parallel with the table. This is Position 1. Bring your wrist towards your thumb. This is Position 2. Return to Position 1.

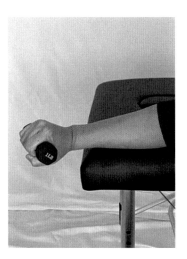

Position 2

When you return to Position 1, this completes one repetition of this exercise. This exercise is to strengthen the muscles on the forearm between the wrist and elbow on the thumb side.

Repeat exercise 10 times for 1 set. Take a break between sets. Aim to perform 3 sets. Repeat exercise with other hand. Discontinue if you experience pain.

Wrist Ulna Deviation

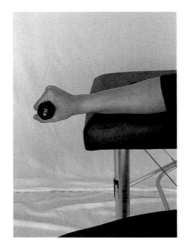

Position 1

Sit down on a chair. Place your forearm on a table or bed, with the wrist hanging off the edge.

The wrist should be parallel with the table. This is Position 1. Bring your wrist towards your pinky (5th digit)

This is Position 2. Return to Position 1.

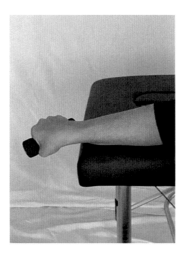

Position 2

When you return to Position 1, this completes one repetition of this exercise.

This exercise is to strengthen the muscles on the forearm between the wrist and elbow on the pinky (5th digit) side. Repeat exercise 10 times for 1 set. Take a break between sets.

Aim to perform 3 sets. Repeat exercise with other hand. Discontinue if you experience pain.

Wrist Supination

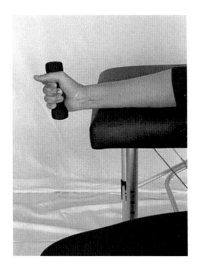

Position 1

Sit down on a chair. Place your forearm on a table or bed, with the wrist hanging off the edge.

The wrist should be perpendicular with the table. This is Position 1. Rotate your palm to face upwards.

Make sure you are rotating your forearm only and not your shoulder. This is Position 2. Return to Position 1.

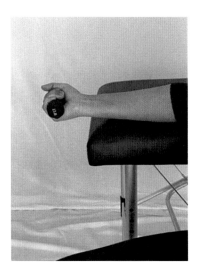

Position 2

When you return to Position 1, this completes one repetition of this exercise. This exercise is to strengthen the muscles in the forearm that help rotate your wrist. Repeat exercise 10 times for 1 set. Take a break between sets. Aim to perform 3 sets. Repeat exercise with other hand. Discontinue if you experience pain.

Wrist Pronation

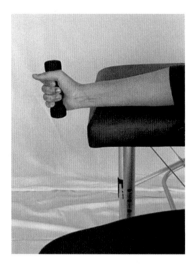

Position 1

Sit down on a chair. Place your forearm on a table or bed, with the wrist hanging off the edge. The wrist should be perpendicular with the table. This is Position 1. Rotate your palm to face downwards. Make sure you are rotating your forearm only and not your shoulder. This is Position 2. Return to Position 1.

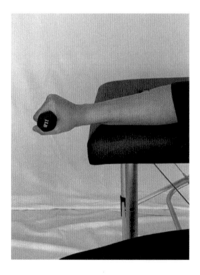

Position 2

When you return to Position 1, this completes one repetition of this exercise. This exercise is to strengthen the muscles in the forearm that help rotate your wrist. Repeat exercise 10 times for 1 set. Take a break between sets. Aim to perform 3 sets. Repeat exercise with other hand. Discontinue if you experience pain.

Grip Strengthening

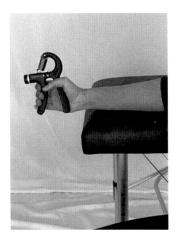

Position 1

Sit down on a chair. Place your forearm on a table or bed, with the wrist hanging off the edge.

The wrist should be perpendicular with the table. Hold stress ball or grip strengthening device in hand. This is Position 1. In Position 1, squeeze stress ball or grip strengthening device. Hold for 2-3 seconds. This is Position 2. Return to Position 1.

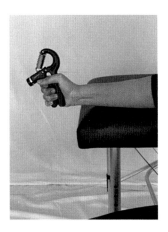

Position 2

When you return to Position 1, this completes one repetition of this exercise. This exercise is to strengthen the muscles on the hand and forearm that allow your hand to grip objects. Repeat exercise 10 times for 1 set. Take a break between sets. Aim to perform 3 sets. Repeat exercise with other hand. Discontinue if you experience pain.

Wrist Extensor Stretch

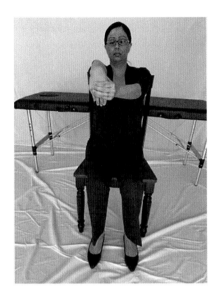

Sitting Position

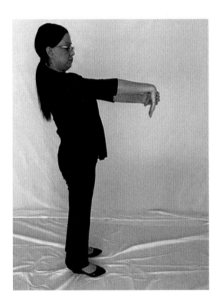

Standing Position

This stretch can be performed in either sitting or standing position. Extend your arm fully at shoulder level. Bring your wrist down using your opposite hand until you feel a stretch.

You should feel a stretch on the top of your forearm. Hold for 10 – 20 seconds. Relax stretch for 10-20 seconds. Repeat this stretch 2-3 times. Repeat the above stretch in the opposite arm. Discontinue stretch if you experience pain

Wrist Flexor Stretch

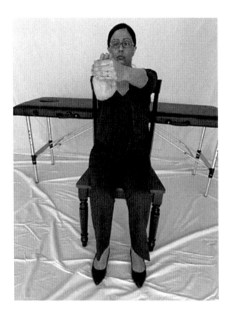

Sitting Position

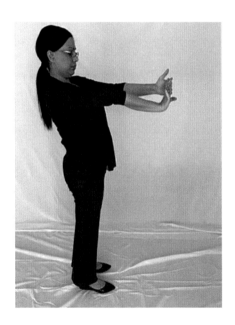

Standing Position

This stretch can be performed in either sitting or standing position. Extend your arm fully at shoulder level. Bring your wrist up using your opposite hand until you feel a stretch. You should feel a stretch on the bottom of your forearm. Hold for 10 – 20 seconds. Relax stretch for 10-20 seconds. Repeat this stretch 2-3 times. Repeat the above stretch in the opposite arm. Discontinue stretch if you experience pain

Shoulder Stretch #1

<u>This stretch should not be performed if you have a history of shoulder dislocation or surgery.</u>

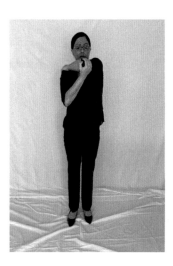

Position 1

Stand upright without slouching. Raise your arm to shoulder level. Bend your elbow. Place your opposite hand on elbow. This is Position 1. Bring your shoulder across your chest using your opposite arm. This is Position 2. This stretch should be felt in your shoulder.

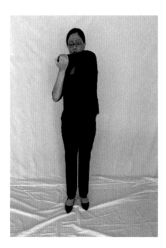

Position 2

Hold for 10 – 20 seconds. Relax stretch for 10-20 seconds. Repeat this stretch 2-3 times. Repeat the above stretch in the opposite arm. Discontinue stretch if you experience pain.

Shoulder Stretch #2

<u>This stretch should not be performed if you have a history of shoulder dislocation or surgery.</u>

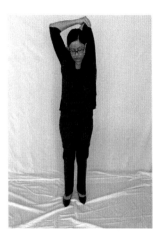

Position 1

Stand upright without slouching. Raise your arm over your head. Bend your elbow. Place your opposite hand on elbow. This is Position 1. Use your opposite hand to bring your elbow up and over your head. This is Position 2. This stretch should be felt in your shoulder.

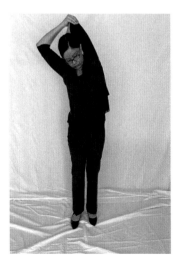

Position 2

Hold for 10 – 20 seconds. Relax stretch for 10-20 seconds. Repeat this stretch 2-3 times. Repeat the above stretch in the opposite arm. Discontinue stretch if you experience pain.

Corner Pectoralis Stretch

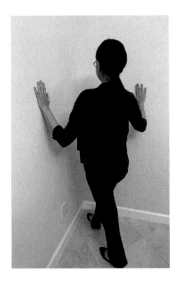

Position 1

Stand at a corner with forearms against wall. Do not shrug your shoulders. Keep your hands below shoulder level. One foot should be placed in front. This is Position 1. Lean forward until you feel a stretch in your chest. This is Position 2.

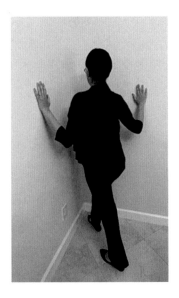

Position 2

Hold for 10 – 20 seconds. Relax stretch for 10-20 seconds. Repeat this stretch 2-3 times. Discontinue stretch if you experience pain.

Door Post Stretch

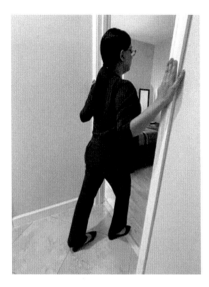

Position 1

Stand at a doorframe with forearms against doorposts. Do not shrug your shoulders. Keep your hands at shoulder level. One foot should be placed in front. This is Position 1. Lean forward until you feel a stretch in your chest. This is Position 2.

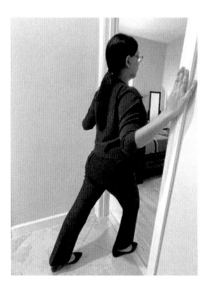

Position 2

Hold for 10 – 20 seconds. Relax stretch for 10-20 seconds. Repeat this stretch 2-3 times. Discontinue stretch if you experience pain.

Upper Trapezius Stretch

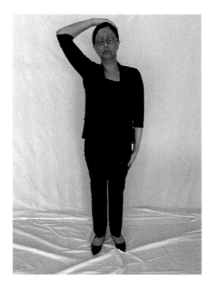

Position 1

Stand upright without slouching. Raise your arm and place your hand on the opposite side of your head. This is Position 1. Gently bend your neck by bringing your ear to your shoulder. This is Position 2. You should feel this stretch on the side of your neck and upper shoulder.

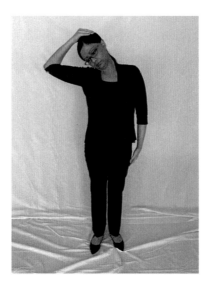

Position 2

Hold for 10 – 20 seconds. Relax stretch for 10-20 seconds. Repeat this stretch 2-3 times. Repeat stretch on the opposite side. Discontinue stretch if you experience pain.

CHAPTER 5:

INTRODUCTION TO LOWER BACK EXERCISES

Introduction to Lumbar Spine (Lower Back)

The lumbar spine (lower back) consists of 5 vertebrae. Vertebrae are the bones that hold the weight of the lower back. In between the vertebrae are the intervertebral discs. They function as shock absorbers for the lumbar spine.

The spinal cord is located inside the vertebrae. The spinal cord in the lower back contains nerves that go into the legs. The nerves that go into the legs can get injured in the lower back or along the path they travel into the legs. The spinal cord and nerves can also be pinched by the intervertebral disc being pushed out of position (also known as a disc herniation).

Muscle spasms (knots in muscle) or tightness occur in the muscles around the lower back and legs. Muscle spasms or tightness in the lower back and legs can also increase pain and limit motion. Muscle spasms can decrease flexibility and cause poor posture. Stretching is helpful to increase flexibility and improve posture.

Poor posture in the lower back can cause the vertebrae to be in poor alignment. This poor alignment can cause muscle weakness or tightness. When the muscles are weak or tight, there is an increased risk of lower back pain or injury. Exercises and stretches are helpful to strengthen weak muscles, stretch tight muscles, improve posture and prevent re-injury.

CHAPTER 6:

LOWER BACK FIRST PHASE

Lower Back First Phase

The First Phase of injury describes the initial injury or pain caused by events such as a fall, car accident or lifting something heavy. The First Phase of an injury can typically last 1-2 weeks depending on the severity of the injury. The areas that are injured are very sensitive to touch. In addition, swelling and redness may also be seen. During this phase, treatment such as medications, rest and ice may be helpful to decrease pain and prevent further injury. <u>Treatment during initial injury should be underneath a physician's supervision.</u>

The pain associated with the initial injury can be decreased with the above treatment. Gentle massage therapy can be used to decrease muscle tightness. <u>Massage therapy should be initiated after consultation with a physician.</u> Once a person is no longer in pain, then gentle therapeutic exercises can be implemented. Exercises in this phase are performed lying down. Exercises should be performed on a bed and **not** on the floor. When performing exercises be sure to breathe normally. Do not hold your breath.

<u>Before beginning any exercise therapy, it is important to consult your physician and make sure these exercises are appropriate for you.</u> Exercises should not be performed if there is any pain. If there is any pain when exercising, discontinue exercise and see a physician.

Lower Back First Phase Exercises and Stretches

Single Knee to Chest Stretch – the purpose of this stretch is to stretch the muscles in the lower back to decrease pain and improve flexibility. <u>**This stretch should not be performed if you have a history of hip dislocation or hip surgery.**</u>

Active Hamstring Stretch (Lying down) – the purpose of this stretch is to stretch the muscles in the back of the leg and improve flexibility. <u>**This stretch should not be performed if you have a history of hip dislocation or hip surgery.**</u>

Abdominal Strengthening/Finding Neutral Pelvis – the purpose of this exercise is to strengthen the muscles in the abdomen. The neutral pelvis is the best position for spinal alignment.

Pelvic Tilts – the purpose of this exercise is to strengthen the muscles in the abdomen to support the lower back.

Glut Sets – the purpose of this exercise is to strengthen the muscles in the buttock. Strengthening the muscles in this region helps support the lower back.

Hip Adduction - the purpose of this exercise is to strengthen the muscles on the inside of the thigh. Strengthening the muscles in this region helps support the lower back.

Hamstring Isometric Strengthening - the purpose of this exercise is to strengthen the muscles on the back of the upper thigh. Strengthening the muscles in this region helps support the lower back.

Clam Shells (Side lying Hip Abduction) - the purpose of this exercise is to strengthen the muscles on the outside of the upper thigh. Strengthening the muscles in this region helps support the lower back. <u>**This exercise should not be performed if you have a history of hip dislocation or hip surgery.**</u>

Seated Knee Extension - the purpose of this exercise is to strengthen the muscles on the front of the thigh. Strengthening the muscles in this region helps support the lower back.

Seated Toe Raises - the purpose of this exercise is to strengthen the muscles in the front of the lower leg. Strengthening the muscles in this region helps support the lower back.

Seated Calf Raises - the purpose of this exercise is to strengthen the muscles in the back of the lower leg. Strengthening the muscles in this region helps support the lower back.

Single Knee to Chest

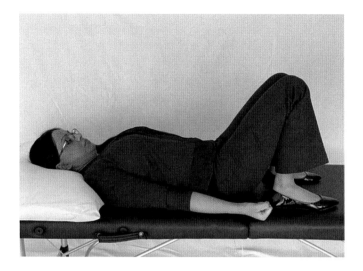

Position 1

<u>This stretch should not be performed if you have a history of hip dislocation or hip surgery.</u>

Lay on your back with your knees bent. This is Position 1. Bring one knee to your chest by grasping your hand under your thigh. Keep the opposite knee in a bent position to support your lower back. This is Position 2. You should feel a stretch in your lower back.

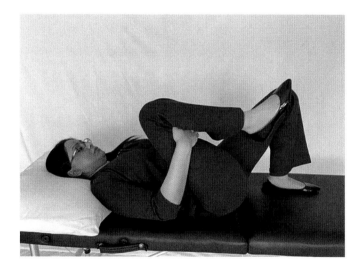

Position 2

Hold for 10 – 20 seconds. Relax stretch for 10-20 seconds. Repeat this stretch 2-3 times.

Repeat the above stretch in the opposite leg. Discontinue stretch if you experience pain.

Active Hamstring Stretch (Lying down)

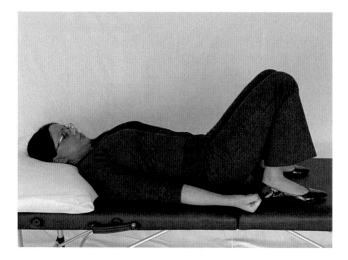

Position 1

This stretch should not be performed if you have a history of hip dislocation or hip surgery.

Lay on your back with your knees bent. This is Position 1. Bring one knee to your chest by grasping your hand under your thigh. Straighten your leg until stretch is felt in the back of the thigh. Keep the opposite knee in a bent position to support your lower back. This is Position 2. You should feel a stretch in the back of the leg.

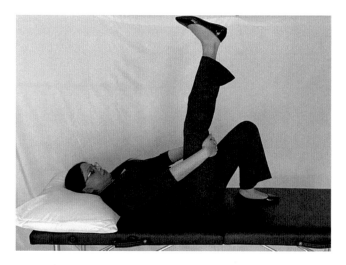

Position 2

Hold for 10 – 20 seconds. Relax stretch for 10-20 seconds. Repeat this stretch 2-3 times. Repeat the above stretch in the opposite leg. Discontinue stretch if you experience pain.

Abdominal Strengthening

Finding Your Neutral Pelvis

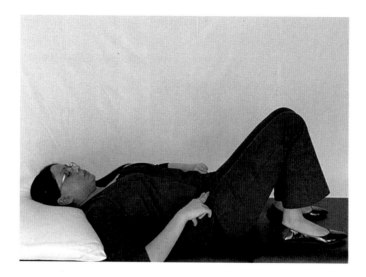

Lay on your back and bend both of your knees. Then tilt your pelvis back all the way, which flattens your back (also known as posterior pelvic tilt). Then tilt your pelvis all the way forward, which arches your back (also known as anterior pelvic tilt). Then position your pelvis in between these two extremes, this is your neutral pelvis.

This is the position your pelvis should be in for normal postural alignment. The exercises will need to be done by holding this position. If you lose this position, you must stop the exercise and try to find it again. Discontinue if you experience pain.

Pelvic Tilts

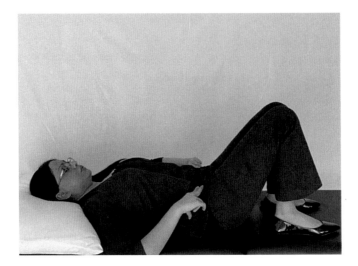

Position 1

Lay on your back and bend both of your knees. This is Position 1. Tilt your pelvis to the neutral pelvis position (refer to the prior page regarding instructions on finding neutral pelvis). This exercise is used to strengthen the abdominal muscles. Place your two fingers on abdomen to feel the muscle tightening with this exercise. This is Position 2. Return to Position 1.

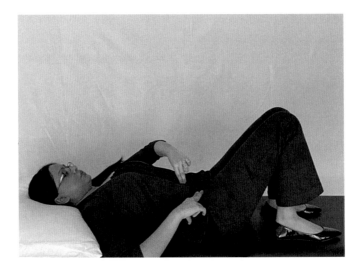

Position 2

When you return to Position 1, this completes one repetition of this exercise. Repeat exercise 10 times for 1 set. Take a break between sets. Aim to perform 3 sets. Discontinue if you experience pain

Glut Sets

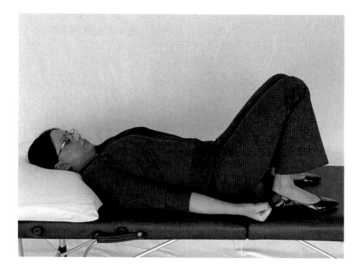

Position 1

Lay on your back with your knees bent. This is Position 1. Squeeze the muscles in the buttock region. Use your fingertips to feel the muscles in your buttock tightening. Hold for 2-3 seconds. This is Position 2. Relax the muscles of the buttock region and return to Position 1.

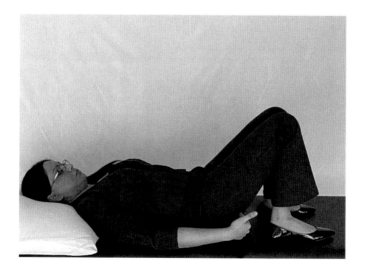

Position 2

When you return to Position 1, this completes one repetition of this exercise. This exercise is used to strengthen the muscles in your buttocks. Repeat exercise 10 times for 1 set. Take a break between sets. Aim to perform 3 sets. Discontinue if you experience pain

Hip Adduction

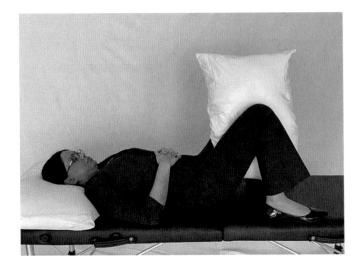

Position 1

Lay on your back with your knees bent. Place a pillow between your legs. This is Position 1.

Squeeze your legs together. Hold for 2-3 seconds. You should feel the muscles on the inside of your thigh

squeezing. This is Position 2. Relax the muscles of the legs and return to Position 1.

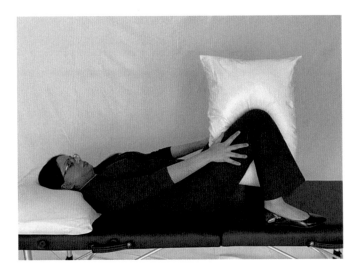

Position 2

When you return to Position 1, this completes one repetition of this exercise. This exercise is used to

strengthen the muscles in the inner thigh. Repeat exercise 10 times for 1 set. Take a break between sets.

Aim to perform 3 sets. Discontinue if you experience pain

Hamstring Isometric Strengthening

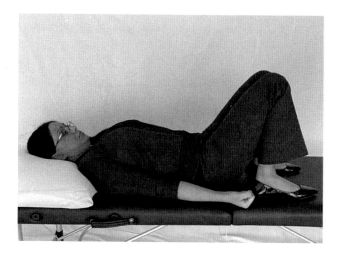

Position 1

Lay on your back with your knees bent. Keep one knee bent to support your lower back.

This is Position 1. Push the opposite heel into the bed. Hold for 2-3 seconds.

You can use your fingertips to feel the muscles tightening in the back of thigh. This is Position 2.

Stop pushing heel into bed and return to Position 1.

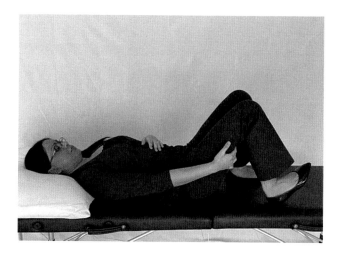

Position 2

When you return to Position 1, this completes one repetition of this exercise. This exercise is used to strengthen the muscles on the back of the thigh. Repeat exercise 10 times for 1 set. Take a break between sets. Aim to perform 3 sets. Repeat the above exercises with the opposite leg. Discontinue if you experience pain.

Clam Shells (Side lying Hip Abduction)

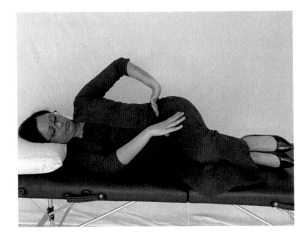

Position 1

<u>**This exercise should not be performed if you have a history of hip dislocation or hip surgery.**</u>

Lay on your side with your knees bent. This is Position 1. Place your hand on your hip to prevent hip and back rotation. Lift your knee up slightly while keeping your ankles together. This is Position 2. Return to Position 1.

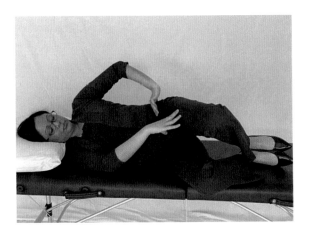

Position 2

When you return to Position 1, this completes one repetition of this exercise. This exercise is used to strengthen the muscles on the outside of the thigh. Repeat exercise 10 times for 1 set.

Take a break between sets. Aim to perform 3 sets. Lay on the opposite side and repeat the above exercises with the opposite leg. Discontinue if you experience pain.

Seated Knee Extension

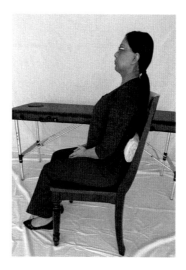

Position 1

Sit upright in a chair with feet on floor. Place a lumbar back roll behind the lower back (for back support).

This is Position 1. Extend your leg straight out in front of you. Hold for 2-3 seconds.

This is Position 2. You should feel the muscles on the front of the thigh tightening. Return to Position 1.

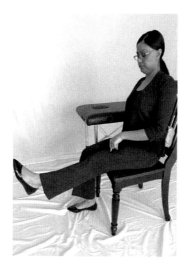

Position 2

When you return to Position 1, this completes one repetition of this exercise. This exercise is used to strengthen the muscles on the front of the thigh. Repeat exercise 10 times for 1 set. Take a break between sets. Aim to perform 3 sets. Repeat exercise with opposite leg. Discontinue if you experience pain.

Seated Toe Raises

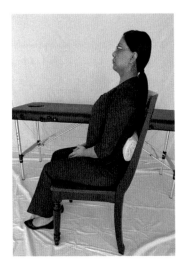

Position 1

Sit upright in a chair with feet on floor. Place lumbar back roll behind the lower back (for back support). This is Position 1. With your heels on the floor, lift both feet upward. This is Position 2. You should feel the muscles on the front of the lower leg tightening. Return to Position 1.

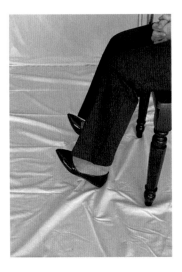

Position 2

When you return to Position 1, this completes one repetition of this exercise. This exercise is used to strengthen the muscles on the front of the lower leg. Repeat exercise 10 times for 1 set.

Take a break between sets. Aim to perform 3 sets. Discontinue if you experience pain.

Seated Calf Raises

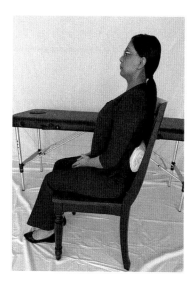

Position 1

Sit upright in a chair with feet on floor. Place lumbar back roll behind the lower back (for back support). This is Position 1. With your toes on the floor, lift both heels upward. This is Position 2. You should feel the muscles on the back of the lower leg tightening. Return to Position 1.

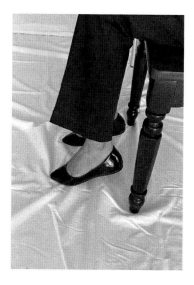

Position 2

When you return to Position 1, this completes one repetition of this exercise. This exercise is used to strengthen the muscles on the back of the lower leg. Repeat exercise 10 times for 1 set. Take a break between sets. Aim to perform 3 sets. Discontinue if you experience pain.

CHAPTER 7:

LOWER BACK SECOND PHASE

Lower Back Second Phase

The Second Phase of injury is when the person is not experiencing much pain. However, the person is weak and is at risk for re-injury. The exercises and stretches in this phase should not be performed if there is any pain or discomfort. Continue exercises and stretches from Lower Back First Phase unless specified below.

Neutral Pelvis with Hip Lift – This exercise is a progression of the Pelvic Tilts in the First Phase. The purpose of this exercise is to strengthen the muscles in the abdomen. Strengthening the muscles in this region helps support the lower back. If you can perform this exercise without pain, you can discontinue Pelvic Tilts from the First Phase.

Seated Hip Flexion - the purpose of this exercise is to strengthen the muscles in the front of the hip. Strengthening the muscles in this region helps support the lower back. **This exercise should not be performed if you have a history of hip dislocation or hip surgery.**

Seated Knee Extension- the purpose of this exercise is to strengthen the muscles in the front of the thigh. Strengthening the muscles in this region helps support the lower back.

Seated Hip Adduction- this exercise is a progression of the Lying Down Hip Adduction in the First Phase. The purpose of this exercise is to strengthen the muscles of the inner thigh.

Strengthening the muscles in this region helps support the lower back. If you can perform this exercise, you can discontinue Lying Down Hip Adduction from the First Phase.

Bridges - this exercise is a progression of the Glut Sets in the First Phase. The purpose of this exercise is to strengthen muscles in the buttock region. Strengthening the muscles in this region helps support the lower back.

Seated Hamstring Stretch - This stretch is a progression of the Lying Down Hamstring Stretch in the First Phase. The purpose of this stretch is to stretch the muscles in the back of the leg and improve flexibility. If you can perform this stretch, you can discontinue Lying Down Hamstring Stretch from the First Phase. **This stretch should not be performed if you have a history of hip dislocation or hip surgery.**

Seated Calf Stretch - the purpose of this stretch is to stretch the muscles in the back of the lower leg and improve flexibility. **This stretch should not be performed if you have a history of hip dislocation or hip surgery.**

Neutral Pelvis with Hip Lift

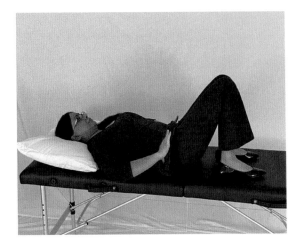

Position 1

Lay on your back and bend both of your knees. This is Position 1. Tilt your pelvis to the neutral pelvis position (see the prior chapter for instructions regarding finding neutral pelvis). Hold neutral pelvis position. Then lift your leg 2 to 4 inches from bed. This exercise is used to strengthen the abdominal muscles. Place your two fingers on abdomen to feel the muscle tightening with this exercise. This is Position 2. Return to Position 1.

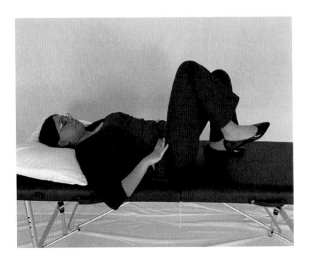

Position 2

When you return to Position 1, this completes one repetition of this exercise. Repeat exercise 10 times for 1 set. Take a break between sets. Aim to perform 3 sets. Repeat exercise on opposite side. Discontinue if you experience pain.

Seated Hip Flexion

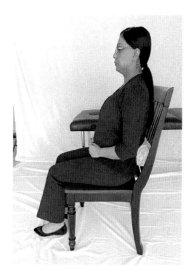

Position 1

<u>This exercise should not be performed if you have a history of hip dislocation or hip surgery.</u>

Sit upright in a chair with feet on floor. Place lumbar back roll behind the lower back (for back support). This

is Position 1. Raise your hip. This is Position 2. You should feel the muscles on the front of the hip tightening.

This exercise is used to strengthen the muscles on the front of the hip. Return to Position 1.

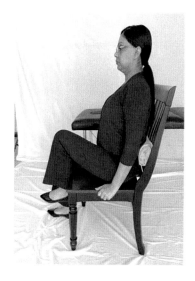

Position 2

When you return to Position 1, this completes one repetition of this exercise. Repeat exercise 10 times for

1 set. Take a break between sets. Aim to perform 3 sets. Repeat exercise with opposite leg. Discontinue if

you experience pain.

Seated Knee Extension

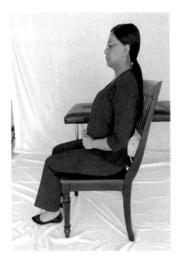

Position 1

Sit upright in a chair with feet on floor. Place lumbar back roll behind the lower back (for back support). This is Position 1. Extend your leg straight out in front of you. Hold for 2-3 seconds. This is Position 2. You should feel the muscles on the front of the thigh tightening. This exercise is used to strengthen the muscles on the front of the thigh. Return to Position 1.

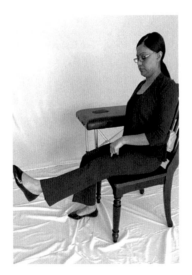

Position 2

When you return to Position 1, this completes one repetition of this exercise. Repeat exercise 10 times for 1 set. Take a break between sets. Aim to perform 3 sets. Repeat exercise on opposite side. Discontinue if you experience pain.

Seated Hip Adduction

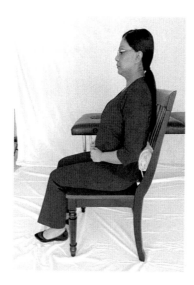

Position 1

Sit upright in a chair with feet on floor. Place lumbar back roll behind the lower back (for back support). This is Position 1. Place pillow between your legs. Squeeze your legs together into the pillow. Hold for 2-3 seconds. This is Position 2. You should feel the muscles on the inside of the thigh tightening. This exercise is used to strengthen the muscles on the inside of the thigh.

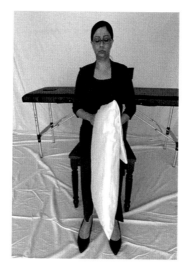

Position 2

Repeat exercise 10 times for 1 set. Take a break between sets. Aim to perform 3 sets. Discontinue if you experience pain.

Bridges

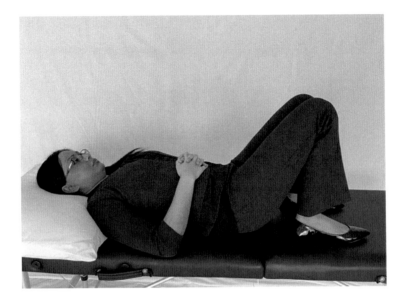

Position 1

Lay on your back with your knees bent. This is Position 1. Lift your buttocks off the bed. Hold for 2-3 seconds. This is Position 2. This exercise is used to strengthen the muscles in your buttocks. Return to Position 1.

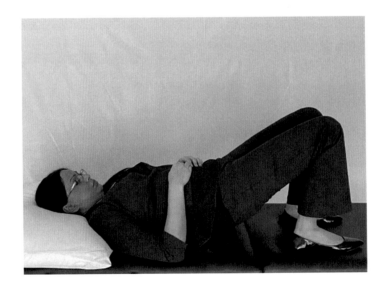

Position 2

When you return to Position 1, this completes one repetition of this exercise. Repeat exercise 10 times for 1 set. Take a break between sets. Aim to perform 3 sets. Discontinue if you experience pain.

Seated Hamstring Stretch

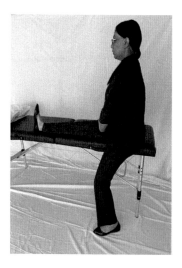

Position 1

<u>This stretch should not be performed if you have a history of hip dislocation or hip surgery.</u>

Sit on the edge of the bed, with one foot on the floor. Keep your back upright. Straighten leg on bed completely. This is Position 1. Lean slightly forward while keeping back straight. This is Position 2. You should feel a stretch in the back of your upper leg.

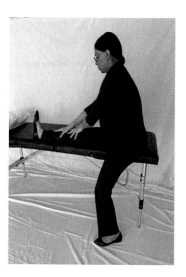

Position 2

Hold for 10 – 20 seconds. Relax stretch for 10-20 seconds. Repeat this stretch 2-3 times.

Repeat the above stretch in the opposite leg. Discontinue stretch if you experience pain.

Seated Calf Stretch

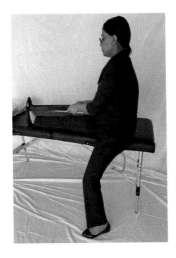

Position 1

<u>This stretch should not be performed if you have a history of hip dislocation or hip surgery.</u>

Sit on the edge of the bed, with one foot on the floor. Keep your back upright. Straighten leg on bed completely. Wrap a belt around your foot. This is Position 1. Using the belt, pull your foot towards yourself. This is Position 2. You should feel a stretch in the back of your lower leg.

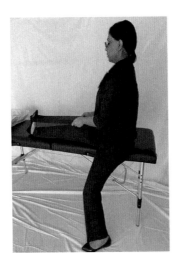

Position 2

Hold for 10 – 20 seconds. Relax stretch for 10-20 seconds. Repeat this stretch 2-3 times.

Repeat the above stretch in the opposite leg. Discontinue stretch if you experience pain.

CHAPTER 8:

LOWER BACK THIRD PHASE

Lower Back Third Phase

The Third Phase of injury is when the person is not experiencing any pain. The exercises and stretches performed in this phase of injury are designed to improve strength and stability of the surrounding joints. Strengthening the muscles of the abdomen and legs can increase stability of the lower back. Stretches in the Third Phase will improve flexibility and will decrease risk of re-injury. Continue exercises and stretches from First and Second Phases unless specified below.

Standing Hip Flexion- the purpose of this exercise is to strengthen the muscles in the front of the hip. Strengthening the muscles in this region helps support the lower back.

Standing Hip Abduction- this exercise is a progression of the Side Lying Hip Abduction (Clam Shells) in the First and Second Phase. The purpose of this exercise is to strengthen the muscles on the outside of the thigh. Strengthening the muscles in this region helps support the lower back. If you can perform this exercise, you can discontinue Side Lying Hip Abduction (Clam Shells) from the First and Second Phases.

Standing Hip Extension- this exercise is a progression of the Bridges in the Second Phase. The purpose of this exercise is to strengthen the muscles in the buttock region. Strengthening the muscles in this region helps support the lower back. If you can perform this exercise, you can discontinue Bridges from the Second Phase.

Standing Hamstring Curls- This exercise is a progression of the Hamstring Isometric Strengthening in the First and Second Phases. The purpose of this exercise is to strengthen muscles in the back of the thigh. Strengthening the muscles in this region helps support the lower back. If you can perform this exercise, you can discontinue Hamstring Isometric Strengthening in the First and Second Phases.

Standing Calf Raises- this exercise is a progression of the Seated Calf Raises in the First and Second Phases. The purpose of this exercise is to strengthen the muscles in the back of the lower leg. Strengthening the muscles in this region helps support the lower back. If you can perform this exercise, you can discontinue Seated Calf Raises in the First and Second Phases.

Mini Squats- the purpose of this exercise is to strengthen the muscles in the buttock and thigh. Strengthening the muscles in this region helps support the lower back.

Quadriceps Stretch- the purpose of this stretch is to stretch the muscles in the front of the thigh. Stretching the muscles in this region helps improve flexibility in the lower back.

Standing Hip Flexion

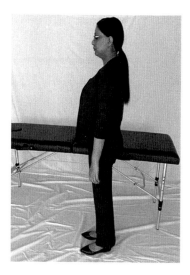

Position 1

Stand upright and hold on to a sturdy surface. This is Position 1. Raise your leg to hip level. This is Position 2. You should feel the muscles on the front of the hip tightening. This exercise is used to strengthen the muscles on the front of the hip. Return to Position 1.

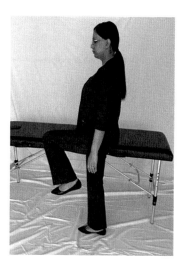

Position 2

When you return to Position 1, this completes one repetition of this exercise. Repeat exercise 10 times for 1 set. Take a break between sets. Aim to perform 3 sets. Repeat exercise on opposite side. Discontinue if you experience pain.

Standing Hip Abduction

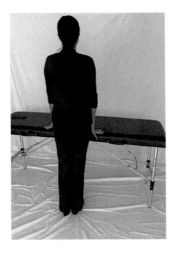

Position 1

Stand upright and hold on to a sturdy surface. This is Position 1. Bring your leg out to your side at a 45-degree angle. This is Position 2. You should feel the muscles on the side of the hip tightening. This exercise is used to strengthen the muscles on the side of the hip.

Return to Position 1.

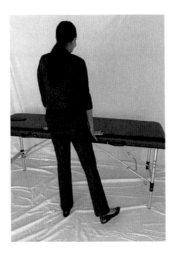

Position 2

When you return to Position 1, this completes one repetition of this exercise. Repeat exercise 10 times for 1 set. Take a break between sets. Aim to perform 3 sets. Repeat exercise on opposite side. Discontinue if you experience pain.

Standing Hip Extension

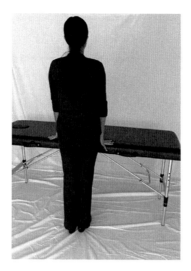

Position 1

Stand upright and hold on to a sturdy surface. This is Position 1. Extend your leg straight behind you. This is Position 2. You should feel the muscles of the buttock and back of your upper leg tightening. This exercise is used to strengthen the muscles of the buttocks and back of the upper leg. Return to Position 1.

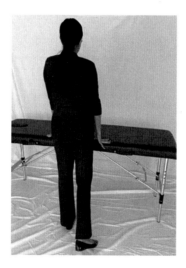

Position 2

When you return to Position 1, this completes one repetition of this exercise. Repeat exercise 10 times for 1 set. Take a break between sets. Aim to perform 3 sets. Repeat exercise on opposite side. Discontinue if you experience pain.

Standing Hamstring Curls

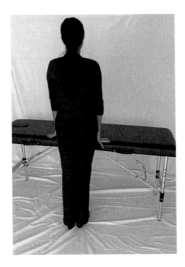

Position 1

Stand upright and hold on to a sturdy surface. This is Position 1. Bend your knee and raise your foot toward your buttocks. This is Position 2. You should feel the muscles on the back of the upper leg tightening. This exercise is used to strengthen the muscles on the back of the upper leg. Return to Position 1.

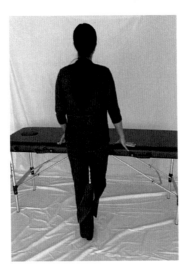

Position 2

When you return to Position 1, this completes one repetition of this exercise. Repeat exercise 10 times for 1 set. Take a break between sets. Aim to perform 3 sets. Repeat exercise on opposite side. Discontinue if you experience pain.

Standing Calf Raises

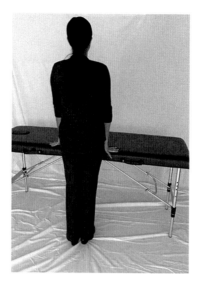

Position 1

Stand upright and hold on to a sturdy surface. This is Position 1. Raise both of your heels as high as tolerated. This is Position 2. You should feel the muscles on the back of the lower leg tightening. This exercise is used to strengthen the muscles on the back of the lower leg. Return to Position 1.

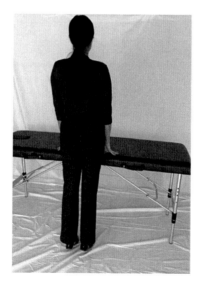

Position 2

When you return to Position 1, this completes one repetition of this exercise. Repeat exercise 10 times for 1 set. Take a break between sets. Aim to perform 3 sets. Discontinue if you experience pain.

Mini Squats

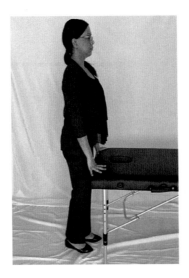

Position 1

Stand upright and hold on to a sturdy surface. Separate your legs to shoulder width apart. This is Position 1. Bend both of your knees and push buttocks region outwards. This is Position 2. You should feel the muscles on the buttock and front/back of upper leg tightening. This exercise is used to strengthen the muscles on the buttock and front/back of upper leg. Return to Position 1.

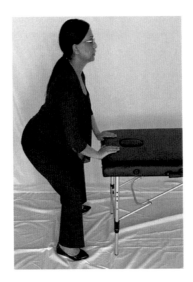

Position 2

When you return to Position 1, this completes one repetition of this exercise. Repeat exercise 10 times for 1 set. Take a break between sets. Aim to perform 3 sets. Discontinue if you experience pain.

Quadriceps Stretch

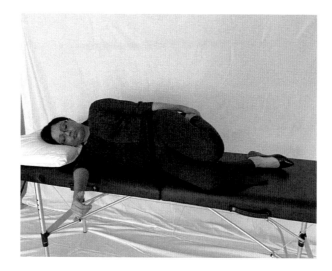

Position 1

This stretch should not be performed if you have a history of hip dislocation or hip surgery. Lay down on your side. The leg on the bottom can be bent slightly (to support the back) or straightened as tolerated. Bend the knee of the leg that is on top. Grasp ankle of leg (with bent knee) with your hand. This is Position 1. Using your hand, gently pull hip and knee backwards as tolerated. This is Position 2. You should feel a stretch in the front of your upper thigh.

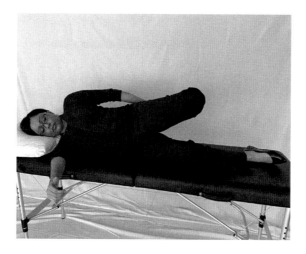

Position 2

Hold for 10 – 20 seconds. Relax stretch for 10-20 seconds. Repeat this stretch 2-3 times. Lay down on opposite side. Repeat the above stretch in the opposite leg. Discontinue stretch if you experience pain.

CHAPTER 9:

TIPS TO DECREASE LOWER BACK PAIN

Tips to Avoid Neck and Lower Back Pain

1. Using a lumbar (lower back) roll when appropriate.

   Reasons why you need a lumbar roll:

   a) Provide support for lower back.

   b) Decrease pain and pressure on the lower back

2. Do not attempt to lift objects that are too heavy for you.

3. Using correct lifting technique when lifting objects.

   a) To decrease pressure on your back, use your legs and keep back as straight as possible.

   b) Wear lumbar brace and appropriate footwear.

4. Use upright posture when performing activities such as brushing teeth and washing dishes.

    a) Keep back as straight as possible.

    b) Avoid bending forward to prevent back pain and re-injury.

5. Use of appropriate sleeping position.

    a) When sleeping on your back, use a pillow underneath your knees to support the lower back.

    b) When sleeping on your side, use a pillow between your knees to support the lower back.

6. Use of proper technique when getting out of bed.

    a) Avoid bending forward when getting out of bed.

How to make a lumbar (lower back) roll

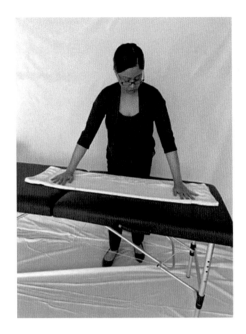

Step 1:

Lay towel unfolded on table and fold towel lengthwise.

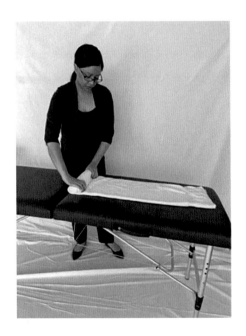

Step 2:

Roll towel.

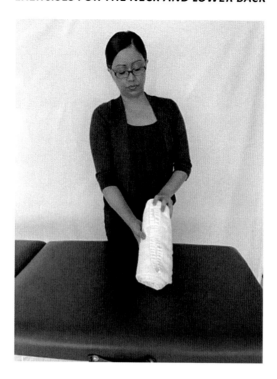

Step 3:

Secure lumbar roll with adhesive tape.

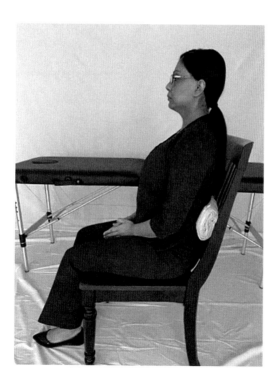

Step 4:

Place lumbar roll behind the curvature of lower back to support the lower back region.

How to lift objects without hurting your back

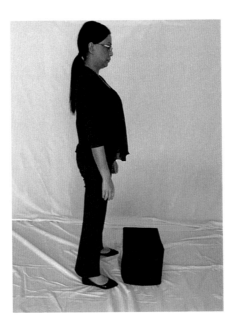

Step 1:

Stand close to the object. Keep feet shoulder length apart. Wear lumbar brace

to support back. Wear appropriate footwear such as sneakers.

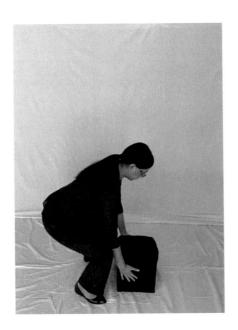

Step 2:

Bend at the knees and stick buttock out to lift object. Keep back straight and avoid bending spine forward.

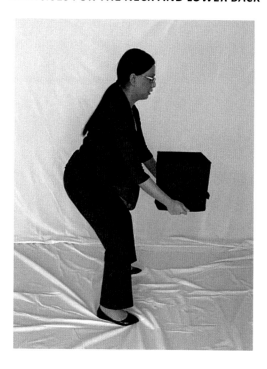

Step 3:

Breathe normally while lifting. Do not hold your breath.

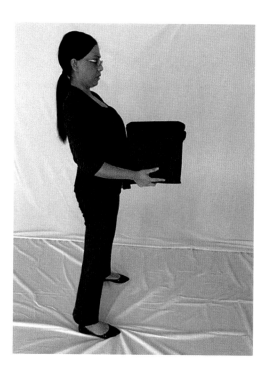

Step 4:

Keep object close to body while lifting.

How to get out of bed without hurting your back

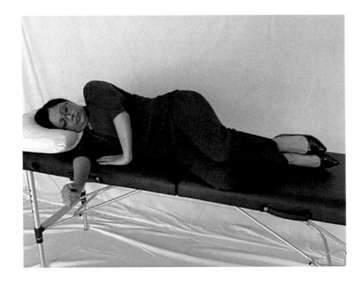

Step 1:

When getting out of bed, first roll over to the side.

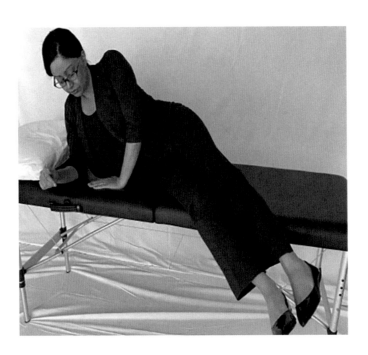

Step 2:

Use hand to push off the bed.

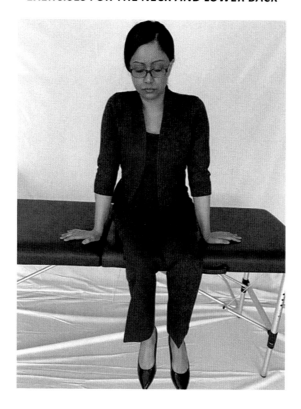

Step 3:

Sit at edge of bed for a few minutes before standing up.

CHAPTER 10:

ACTIVITY MODIFICATION TO DECREASE PAIN

How to brush your teeth without hurting your back

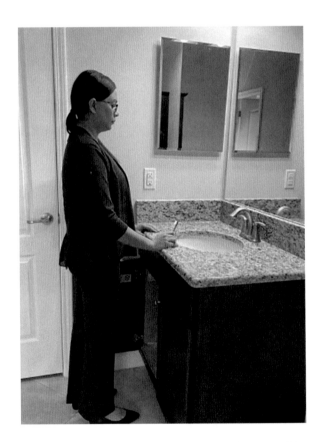

Step 1: Keep back upright. Come close to sink. Open lower cabinet door of sink.

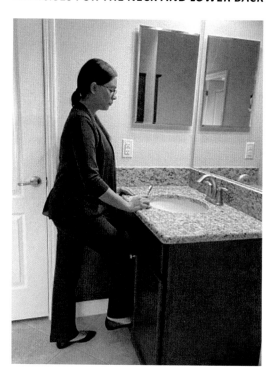

Step 2: Place one foot on the cabinet to give back support.

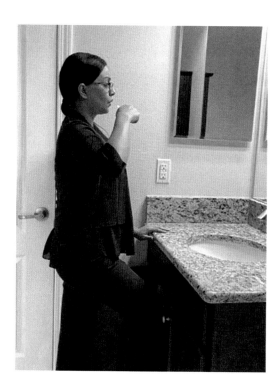

Step 3: Keep back upright and avoid bending forward as much as possible.

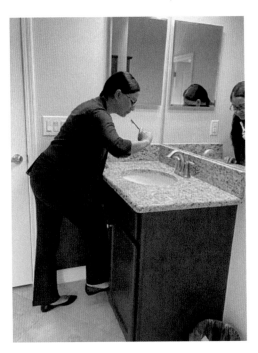

Step 4: Keep back straight and push buttock out when getting closer to sink.

How to wash dishes without hurting your back

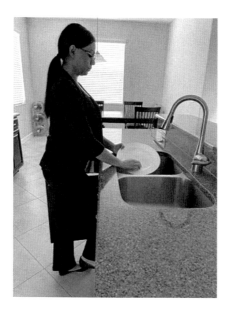

Step 1:

Keep back upright when washing dishes.

Open lower cabinet and place one foot on the cabinet to support back.

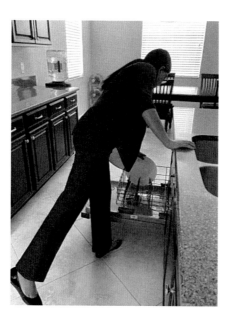

Step 2:

When placing dishes into the dishwasher, use one hand on the counter and

extend leg. Keep back straight to load and unload dishwasher.

How to sleep without hurting your back

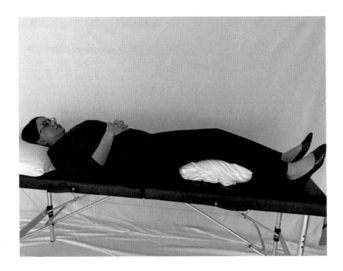

Sleeping on back:

When lying on your back, place pillow underneath your knees to provide lower back support.

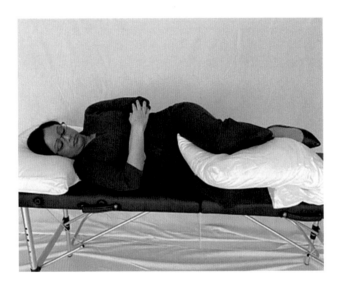

Sleeping on side:

When lying on your side, pillow can be placed between the knees to support back.

CONCLUSION

Exercises and stretches should be continued on a regular basis to prevent re-injury and maintain good posture. Once you can perform all exercises and stretches in Phase 3 without pain, an appropriate cardiovascular exercise regimen (such as light to moderate walking) can be discussed with your physician.

To avoid excessive muscle soreness, exercise 2-3 times a week. An exercise day should be followed by a rest day to allow muscles to heal and recover. Repeat injuries can happen. You can always return to this guide to restore your strength and flexibility. Be sure to follow the protocols as directed.

Thank you for purchasing this book, I hope you found this book helpful. Please share with those who can benefit from this book.

ABOUT THE AUTHOR

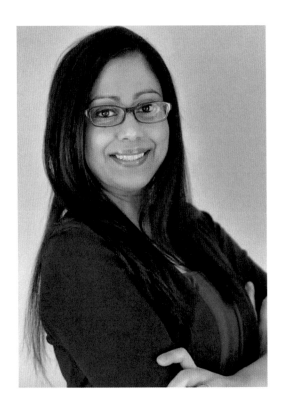

Dr. Sindhu George is a licensed physical therapist. She is a 2005 graduate of New York Institute of Technology with a Doctorate in Physical Therapy (DPT). She has extensive physical therapy experience in outpatient orthopedics, spinal manual therapy and inpatient physical therapy.

Dr. George is the former owner of George Rehabilitation and Wellness, LLC (a physical therapy clinic), where she developed a special interest in the treatment of neck and lower back pain. Dr. George developed a progressive exercise and stretching regimen which led to significant improvement of pain and quality of life for her patients.

Made in the USA
Las Vegas, NV
13 December 2024

14235050R00055